To Gil Lederman:

Thank you for the treatment, and thank you
for having the vision to make it accessible to
people from overseas

Introduction

I began to write this book in 1997 more or less as soon as I returned from treatment. The first draft was well underway by the following year so I sent an outline and the first couple of chapters to a few publishers and received what would politely be called 'encouraging rejection letters'. How can a rejection letter ever be encouraging! They said it was well written but the potential readership was too small to make it a viable proposition. Other people read it and said 'Don't give up, it's very readable and could really help some people.'

So of course I gave up. Other things took over and it remained just another folder on my computer. That is until I stumbled across publishing-on-demand, also known as print-on-demand. No need for a print run; copies could, amazingly, be printed to order one at a time. So I was inspired to find the folder and add a beginning and an end to the story.

The story is my search for a suitable treatment for an uncommon brain tumour; an acoustic neuroma. Conventional medical opinion was that it should be removed surgically, a route that would have left me with one-sided deafness and most likely with facial paralysis as well, other unpleasant side effects were also a distinct possibility. So I refused surgery and searched for a treatment that would deal with the tumour without inflicting injury on the rest of me.

It was a very lonely and difficult journey as friends and family wanted me to follow the advice of the medical experts and have surgery.

As well as acoustic neuroma patients I hope that this book will be helpful to anyone who is facing a really difficult decision. I hope that it's an enjoyable and interesting read, if it's helpful as well then that's even better.

Chapter One

1995

'Did you go to many discos when you were young?' asked the ENT consultant, her eyes never leaving the paper in front of her. Well, I'd been to a few but I took both my ears with me, I don't recall every leaving one of them at home.

'Some degree of high frequency hearing loss is normal at around your age.' She continued.

'So why is only my right ear affected?' I asked. It seemed such a straightforward and obvious question.

'You also do have a lot of wax in your ears.'

'Yes - but I've been told there is more in my left ear and that one's fine.' She looked in both ears, asked me to repeat various words and to walk on the spot with my eyes closed. Yet more questions followed about when symptoms first began and whether there was a history of deafness in the family. She seemed to be ignoring the most obvious features; the distortion and the one-sided nature of the problem. I decided to try to bring her attention to it again.

'What really puzzles me is why my right ear causes music to distort, and why the telephone dialling tone is a different pitch in one ear to the other.'

She suggested a possible cause of the distortion and I felt that at last she seemed to be taking me seriously, to be thinking of things which could be the cause of the problem rather than attempting to dismiss it. Although I didn't fully understand her explanation I understood enough to have what was becoming a familiar response:

'OK, but why is only one ear affected?' I was beginning to get quite exasperated, why was no explanation being put forward?

I could understand why my GP didn't know what the problem was, he had been honest and said I would need to see a hospital consultant. So here I was in a department full of Ear Nose and Throat Specialists and yet I was still not being told the nature of the problem. I found it very difficult to cope with both the nature of the questions and her ignoring of mine. I felt like I was back at the GP surgery again. Somehow this was not corresponding to my expectations of how the appointment would progress. Although I had not consciously thought about it I suppose I must have had some idea as to what the consultation would be like. I had most likely thought that the consultant would list a number of possible causes of my hearing problem, inform me of what tests would be necessary in order to determine the exact cause and suggest treatments. Instead, no causes were being put forward and the most important feature of the problem was apparently being ignored.

One thought kept recurring in my head 'Surely, she must know what the problem is!' If she did she wasn't telling me because every time I asked what might cause something to happen in one ear and not the other I got no response.

What I didn't know at that time, but presumably as an ENT specialist she did, was that I was presenting one of the classic symptoms indicating the presence of an Acoustic Neuroma; one-sided hearing loss. I also now know that by asking me to walk on the spot with my eyes closed she was testing my balance, which at that time was fine. Balance problems are another indication of the presence of an Acoustic Neuroma.

I learned later on that for some people the symptoms associated with Acoustic Neuroma come on very quickly, occasionally almost overnight. In my case that had not happened, the road from the early symptoms to hospital appointment had been a long one. I had first noticed the symptoms some four years previously, starting as an intermittent distortion which was only noticeable when teaching the piano, and even then not all the time. Gradually over the years it had become more frequent and had become apparent in other situations. Although I thought it a nuisance and somewhat unfortunate I wasn't overly concerned, believing it would go away eventually. Maybe that was a rather complacent attitude but it still tends to be my approach to most medical problems; first of all see if it takes care of itself, and gets better. I am definitely not the kind of person who goes rushing off to see the GP at every turn and self-diagnosis books are not my bed-time reading. I also wasn't sure if anything could be done about my hearing problem anyway. I certainly never imagined it could be an indication of a tumour.

It was the telephone dialling tone that finally persuaded me to seek medical advice. I always hold the phone to my left ear and because of that was no doubt unaware as to the extent of hearing loss in my right. One day I put the phone to my right ear and was amazed, and concerned. The pitch of the dialling tone was different. I checked and re-checked but the result was the same – there was a difference of around three notes on the piano between the two. I then thought that perhaps everyone had the same phenomena so I asked my then husband to listen. He heard the same pitch in both ears. I was completely mystified, being totally at a loss to even begin to understand how one ear could hear the same sound at a different pitch to the other one. I also could not understand how the two differing pitches were reconciled when listening to music, or was that the cause of the distortion? On a lighter note I wondered if I'd finally discovered why I had always been completely unable to sing in tune! Even so I still was not unduly alarmed, maybe there was a straightforward explanation. As I had stopped studying biology at school as soon as possible I had no real idea of how the ear worked. One thing was apparent though, even to someone with my laissez faire attitude to health; this problem was not just going to go away, I had to seek medical advice.

A few days after that I saw my GP who looked in my ears for evidence of infection, couldn't find any and booked me in for a hearing test with the nurse. Just in case there was something he couldn't see I was also given a nasal spray and ear drops.

The nurse carried out the hearing test in a consulting room in the surgery. I was given a pair of headphones to wear and asked to indicate when a sound was audible. The sound was a pure tone of various pitches and volumes, sent to each ear in turn. As she said, it wasn't an ideal test because the general noise of the surgery could still be heard in the background, but it would give an indication as to whether or not further investigation was necessary. At the end she showed me the results; a very definite high frequency hearing loss in my right ear. Her opinion was that I would be referred to the ENT clinic at the local hospital, which I duly was.

And so I had arrived at the ENT clinic fully confident that they would be able to tell me the cause of my strange hearing problem, a confidence born of the perception that I was now going to see the experts. On arrival I had been given another hearing test, this time in an eerily soundproofed room. The room was so well soundproofed as to be completely quiet. To go from the bustle of the waiting room into silence was quite odd. The test itself was much more extensive than the one carried out by the nurse. The first part again consisted of indicating when I could hear a tone in each ear, this was followed by listening for a tone in one ear while a masking, rushing sound was played in the other. For another part of the test a different kind of headphone was used and placed on the bone behind the ear. I'm not sure what the different tests were for but I felt that they were so comprehensive that they must provide the necessary information with which to make a diagnosis. The results were sent with me to the consultant.

It was therefore surprising that they did not apparently provide any useful additional information. All the consultant seemed to be doing was agreeing that I had a hearing problem in one ear. I did not need to visit a specialist to be told that.

I knew the consultation was drawing to a close, unsatisfactorily, when she suggested I should have a further hearing test and take some ear drops to get rid of the wax. At that point it seemed as if she didn't know any more than my GP, but I felt that she must. And it was also at that point I felt myself getting annoyed and exasperated. I was beginning to get an overwhelming feeling of 'just why did I come here in the first place!' A GP cannot be expected to have in depth knowledge of every part of the body, which was precisely why I had been referred. These people were specialists, surely they must have some idea of what was wrong? I could not be the first person to be referred with distortion in one ear. Also, she had never actually said that she didn't know what the cause of the problem might be. She had been very evasive but had never actually said 'I don't know, you've got me beat on that one.' Or whatever the equivalent medical speak may be. If she had said something along those lines I would most likely have taken the ear drops and left. Although I cannot actually remember thinking 'She knows more than she's saying' maybe I was in some way aware of the possibility, and it was that awareness which made me feel so frustrated when the only treatment she suggested was exactly that which my GP had already tried.

'My GP gave me a nasal spray and ear drops when I first saw him.' I explained, being aware that I was perhaps now beginning to sound as exasperated as I felt.

'These are much stronger than the ones he would have given you.'

'But I still don't understand why all this is only happening in one ear.' As I spoke she was already writing out the request for another hearing test, along with the prescription for ear drops.

'Well, I suppose we could send you for an MRI scan just to rule out anything more sinister.' she finally conceded.

At last, a test that wasn't a hearing test! I felt as if in a way she had said 'Well I don't know what the problem is but this scan may unearth it.' I wasn't even sure at that time what a MRI scan was or what they were used for, but I knew that scans in general can look at 'things inside' and that was sufficient for me.

It never crossed my mind to ask what the 'something more sinister' might possibly be and it was obvious that she wasn't going to tell me, as by now the nurse was taking away my notes and the prescription was in my hand. However, I was not concerned. I had had enough. I just wanted to be out of the hospital and home as soon as possible. I wanted peace. The whole consultation had been such an ordeal that I was totally incapable of prolonging it by attempting to discover more about the MRI scan and what it nay uncover.

It's said that 'The British' don't like to complain and don't complain enough. That may not be true any more, it may never have been true, but it certainly is true for me as an individual. In my case childhood memories of waiting with my mother while she complained about an item of clothing in Marks and Spencer linger on. I'm sure she was quite right to complain, but I didn't like the fuss then and I still do not like it.

I most certainly viewed medical people as experts, they knew what was best, it was their job. My medical history such as it was, was one of me being a good patient. I did not ask questions other than very polite innocent ones and I did as I was told. In addition I was, and still am, a conflict avoider. Conflict is upsetting, uncomfortable, difficult to get over and therefore to be avoided if at all possible. In short, I'm just like the majority of people; all I want is to be left in peace to get on with my life; if people leave me alone I'll leave them alone.

So what made me different that day? The good patient response would have been to take the prescription for the ear drops and say 'Thank You'. I asked far too many questions and was even impolite enough to keep asking the same one repeatedly. I prolonged the consultation after the point where a good patient would have left. I was not a good patient, but why not?

I think that it was a combination of different factors. Firstly, common sense. Both my ears had always been places together and I had not been given a satisfactory explanation as to why one should behave differently to the other. Secondly, the birth of my son. He was born 10 weeks prematurely and at the time I asked every medical person I met 'What are the possible long term effects of prematurity?' I was constantly reassured that he would be fine, that by the time he was 3 years old he would have caught up lost ground. When he was 18 months old he was diagnosed with Cerebral Palsy and registered disabled. I then discovered that there is a high incidence of Cerebral Palsy among premature babies. The medical people I had asked had avoided telling me something they most certainly knew; that he was at an increased risk of Cerebral Palsy. I'm sure they didn't tell me because they didn't want me to worry, he could have been fine. The down side of them not telling me was that it was much more of a shock, and therefore more difficult to cope with, when he finally was diagnosed than it would have been if I had always known of the possibility. That whole experience must have fundamentally changed my view of medical people and most certainly resulted in a breakdown of trust. I no longer assumed medics would tell me all relevant information, even if I asked for it. During the ENT consultation I did not consciously think 'I've been denied information before therefore I could be denied it again', but I behaved as if I did.

Now, looking back, I can see that my previous trust in the medical profession was somewhat naïve, after all why should they be any different to other professions? Everyone makes mistakes, makes errors of judgements, handles something not so well one day as another. It is the mystique which has been allowed to build up around the profession which perhaps causes us to view them differently and in turn to expect from them standards which we would not expect elsewhere. This mystique must be broken down as it does us, as patients, a disservice, and it places responsibility on the profession which is in excess of what is reasonable. We ourselves must accept some responsibility in making decisions about our own health, in both helping ourselves to stay healthy and in treatment decisions when illness strikes. The two go hand in hand; if we are actively interested in promoting our own health then we will also be actively interested in treating our own ill-health.

But back to the consultation - should I have been told that it may be a tumour causing the problem? The doctor's response would perhaps be that she didn't want to cause unnecessary worry, that Acoustic Neuromas are very rare, that they invariably grow very slowly, that they can take some years before they grow large enough to be life-threatening. Maybe she simply did not want to mention the word 'tumour'? Perhaps she was simply trying to save the expense of an MRI scan? Whatever the reason she obviously did not want to tell me and presumably that is why she was so reluctant to discuss likely causes of my one-sided hearing loss. As it was obvious that it hadn't been caused by exposure to environmental factors such as gunshots, it must have been caused by something going wrong in my ear, and to start discussing likely reasons for that would have inevitably had to include Acoustic Neuroma.

Or it could be that she had strong suspicions a tumour was present but also knew that because my symptoms were slight it would be better for me to not undergo any treatment at that time. If so why didn't she **explain** that to me instead of making decisions on my behalf? Are patients not to be trusted to make the correct decision? If that was her logic then what is worrying is the possibility that she could not trust her own colleagues to refrain from treating a tumour unnecessarily.

So many questions and obviously no answers as I have never seen her again. I would still like to know the answers, but cannot believe anything would convince me that ear drops were really the best course of action to take at that time.

Chapter Two

England

The appointment for the second hearing test came through within a few weeks. The test itself didn't seem very different from the first one and apparently didn't show anything new. When I asked the technician his opinion he was vague, which did not surprise me because I was becoming accustomed to vagueness.

So I waited patiently for the MRI appointment and continued to teach the piano and lead a normal life. The only problem was that some pupils were proving very uncomfortable to teach. The distortion was now accompanied by a pain in the ear and I found myself wanting to say 'Don't play so loudly!', but of course I couldn't! – *Forte* is supposed to be loud. In addition to the pain being triggered by the volume it was also worse with higher pitches than lower ones. Quite a serious effect was that at times the distortion was so bad I actually found it very difficult to hear accurately what the pupil was playing. Attending concerts and listening to music in general were activities that were no longer enjoyable as I simply couldn't hear the music properly. A major part of my life was becoming increasingly absent. Yet the brain is very adaptive. I don't recall thinking 'Oh it would be really nice to be able to go and enjoy a concert,' but I do remember attending concerts and thinking 'I can't hear this properly, it's hurting'. Inevitably that led to an avoidance of the situation and I simply stopped attending concerts. As time progressed it wasn't just concerts that I avoided. The hearing problems made conversations at social events extremely difficult and stressful as I found it very difficult to focus on the voice of the person I was talking; there was so much other noise getting in the way! Even an evening meal with a few friends provided a noise level which caused problems for me, and parties, especially children's parties, were a nightmare. All of this must have meant that my habits changed, but they changed so slowly that I was unaware of them doing so.

I still had absolutely no idea what could be causing it all and neither did anyone else I met. Some people had experience of tinnitus, others knew people who were deaf, but no-one had experience, either directly or indirectly, of distortion and one-sided hearing loss, they were as mystified as I was. To me it felt like something inside my ear had become loose, perhaps it could be re-attached?

As the MRI scan drew closer I was not at all concerned about what it might find. I had no idea of what it might find but I naively assumed it would not be anything very serious. It was the MRI scanner itself that caused more anxiety than anything else. In fact, as I looked at the diagram of the machine I became very concerned that I would panic in some way. Although not claustrophobic as such I have a very real apprehension of being in small lifts, or going underground, so the prospect of being inside a metal tube was not an appealing one. I decided that when the scan was actually in progress I would have to concentrate very hard and imagine I was somewhere relaxing, a mountain or a beach maybe, anywhere but where I actually was. It was therefore those fears that occupied my mind in the days leading up to the scan rather than any concern as to what it might find. Half of me thought that it wouldn't actually find anything and the other half thought that it might, but that it would not be serious.

At that time the local hospital did not have its own scanner, instead, every two weeks one arrived on the back of an articulated lorry. The trailer part contained the scanner itself together with the computing equipment. When I arrived I was given a questionnaire to fill in to confirm that I didn't have any bits of metal that had been left inside after operations or war injuries. Metal from war injuries was not a problem but the likelihood of forgetting about a hair grip was, so I checked and rechecked. The body is a very resilient; I've no idea how strong the magnetic field produced by the scanner is, but it's probably too strong for me to be able to comprehend. Yet the body just accepts it.

The waiting area was very much like the rest of the newly upgraded hospital; a nice carpet on the floor, comfortable chairs and coffee tables with an assortment of magazines. I looked at magazine after magazine but somehow couldn't find one that sustained my interest; perhaps there should have been a copy of 'MRI Scanner To-day!' No doubt there actually is an equivalent trade magazine. My eye caught a notice warning patients that their appointment would be delayed in the event of an emergency and I wondered what kind of emergency they were thinking about. I found out a couple of years later when a friend fell from a mountain and had to be airlifted to the hospital. She was given an MRI to assess the extent of her injuries.

Apparently there were no such incidents that day as although the wait seemed like a long time it was actually only about 30 minutes. About 10 minutes before the scan I was injected with a dye so that the resulting images could be seen more clearly. It was then time to leave the comforting waiting area and go to the scanner. Doing so was an odd experience, being shown out of the waiting area and up the steps of a lorry! That was definitely a first for me. Inside I noticed that the lorry trailer was divided into two parts; the scanner in the main part and the computing equipment in the second. After a brief conversation to check the details I'd provided the nurse took me to the scanner. It looked larger than the one in the picture, but then it was in a very confined space. Seeing the picture first proved to be helpful though as I recognised the sliding table I would lie on. As I tried to make myself comfortable she explained that I would be able to see her and the computer operators by using the 45-degree mirror above my eyes. Very nice, except that it was positioned on a grilled frame which was placed over my face. I felt trapped. The nurse checked that I was comfortable and requested I stay as still as possible while the machine was working. She concluded by recommending that I close my eyes as the table was slid into the machine, and then open them once inside, so that I could watch them in the mirror. She made one final check and then pressed the slide button.

My first thought as the table slid in was how narrow the tube actually was, much narrower than I had expected. I am not a large person but even so both shoulders caught the side. Remembering the nurse's advice I closed my eyes, but even with my eyes closed I could tell that I was going into somewhere darker, which was rather scary. When the table stopped I opened my eyes and looked in the mirror. I could indeed see the staff in the other room operating the equipment. However, I could also see the top of the tube and realised that I was very close to it. Far too close for comfort, maybe 2 inches away, perhaps even less. Furthermore I could also see the grill which was positioned over my face. I felt myself starting to panic so quickly closed my eyes again.

Seeing the grill and the top of the tube caused many thoughts to flash through my mind very quickly. The overriding one was that I had to get out of that tube. I would call them and they would come and slide me back out. But what if the table got stuck and they couldn't get me out? What if they didn't hear me? After all, they were the other side of a glass partition. I had to force myself to remember what I had previously decided to do. There was no point in calling them to get me out of the machine; I would just have to go back in again or wait for another appointment. This was just something I was going to have to do. After all it wasn't going to take long and then I could go back outside to the sunshine.

Having my eyes shut was far preferable. With my eyes shut I couldn't see just how close I was to the top of the tube, my shoulders could still feel the sides but that was much easier to deal with. Slowly the panic began to subside and with no visual image in my mind I could imagine I was elsewhere. Or rather, I could try to imagine I was elsewhere, but those machines are noisy, so noisy as to make it impossible to not be fully aware of their presence. There is an almost constant very loud banging noise, as if someone is on the outside of the tube with a hammer and they're hitting directly around your head. It's a very rhythmical noise, and the pitch does change but it is very, very loud. The only moments of quiet come when the magnet is being moved to a new position, or when the staff are 'stopping to think' (I assume). I'd never known a beach quite that noisy!

I also remembered the antenatal breathing exercises and they really helped. I've found the breathing exercises learned while expecting my first child have been useful in a wide range of situations and this was certainly one of them. I can still remember the midwife's calming voice as she went through the sequence of exercises. So I forced myself to ignore where I was and concentrated on imagining I was back at the health centre surrounded by pregnant women!

Slowly I began to calm down and the sense of panic subsided. It was hard work to keep my thoughts focused, but it worked. Eventually I felt the table sliding back out again, relief, I'd actually managed it! I hadn't panicked or behaved like a small child, the whole process had gone very smoothly. On the way out an appointment was made to get the scan results in two weeks.

For that appointment I saw a different member of the ENT team. This time there were no questions about attending disco's, the doctor got straight to the point:

'You had your MRI two weeks ago and it has shown something. It's very small and if it were anywhere else in the body would not cause any problems, but because it's in a confined space, it is. Unfortunately we don't treat them here so you'll be referred to a large city hospital in England, they know what to do with these cases.'

Chapter Two

I was completely taken aback by the news. I really hadn't expected the scan to have revealed something serious enough to have to go to England for!

'These things are always benign but have to be surgically removed,' he continued 'years ago it used to be a major operation but now it's quite straightforward.' I was really struggling to recover my thoughts and not succeeding very well. I was going to have to have surgery to my head! To remove what exactly? How were they going to remove it? How were they going to get into my head? Why couldn't they perform the operation here? How long would it take to recover? Exactly what did the operation entail? However, while my mind was working very slowly as it tried to take in the information the doctor's was having no such problems. As I tried to assimilate the news he was gathering up my case notes and rushing me out of the room. I tried to ask questions but was told to wait until I saw the experts in England. He gave me the name of someone to phone if I didn't get the appointment within 3 weeks. My notes were gathered together, the doctor was on his feet, the consultation was over. The whole consultation probably took 5 minutes, or even less.

As I was driving home from the hospital I realised that I had not actually been told what 'it' was. It was not that the doctor had told me the name and I had forgotten, he had simply said that it was some sort of growth. But what kind of growth? I had no idea but I did not for a moment think that it was a 'tumour'. I assumed that if it were a tumour I would have been told so. Instead I thought it possibly was like a ganglion, which was the only non-tumour growth I had any experience of. I'd had a ganglion on my wrist and could see how such a growth could cause problems in a confined space. But was it possible for ganglions to grow in the head? I had absolutely no idea.

And where exactly was 'it'? And how would they get 'it' out? I felt very annoyed with myself. I should have asked! I should have asked the questions but was too taken aback. I had needed time to think, not long - just a couple of minutes would have been enough. I simply had not been able to take in the news that the MRI had revealed a growth quickly enough to be able to ask questions. By the time I'd thought of the questions and was able to ask them the doctor was on his feet making a beeline for the door, he had used the time lag to get me out of the room. He obviously did not want to have to talk to me about the nature of the growth, the treatment, the recovery time, or anything. He just wanted to get me out of the room as fast as he could.

My knowledge of anatomy is only marginally greater than that which can be learned from the children's song 'Head, Shoulders, Knees and Toes', so my first stop was the Public Library to look up 'The Ear'. In the pre-internet days information was still the preserve of books. In the books I found diagrams of the ear and its connections to the brain, but nowhere could I find mention of 'it'. I looked up diseases of the ear but still could not find 'it'. I found a myriad of interesting facts about the ear. I learned that the ear consists of three parts; the outer ear, the middle ear and the inner ear. That sound causes the ear drum to vibrate before it passes through the middle ear via tiny bones called *ossicles*. From there it reaches the inner ear which is filled with fluid and the movement of the fluid stimulates the hair cells which trigger a nerve impulse which is carried by the auditory nerve to the brain. Amazingly, once received by the brain it makes sense! It was obviously a very intricate and delicate process and I could see how a growth anywhere could interfere and cause problems. But nowhere could I find mention of 'things that grow in the ear'. I was obviously in need of help. Whatever 'it' was, the GCSE syllabus didn't include 'it'.

So armed with diagrams of various bits of the head I went to see my GP. Thankfully he was very helpful, answering my questions and even showing me the letter he'd received about me. Now I knew what 'it' was; an Acoustic Neuroma. I knew where 'it' was growing; on the auditory nerve in the auditory canal. I knew how big 'it' was; about 1cm long and 5mm wide. The only question he wasn't sure about was how they got 'it' out! However I felt much better after seeing him as armed with the information he'd given me I could easily find out more.

As well as teaching the piano part-time in the University Music Department I was also studying part-time for a PhD so had access to on-line databases. These databases are divided into different subject areas and contain information on articles published in Academic Journals throughout the world. I headed straight for Medline to look up 'Acoustic Neuroma'.

I was about to get a second unpleasant surprise as what I discovered about Acoustic Neuromas did not make pleasant reading. First of all I discovered that the auditory canal serves as an anatomical Spaghetti Junction. A lot of nerves have to pass from various parts of the head through to the brain and the auditory canal provides a ready-made channel through the skull.

Together there are eight of them, collectively called the Cranial Nerves. The auditory nerve, facial nerve and vestibular nerve (responsible for balance) are among the eight and they all lie in close proximity to each other. I learned that some people thought 'it' should be called a Vestibular Schwanoma rather than an Acoustic Neuroma as it usually grows on the vestibular nerve rather than the auditory.

But I wasn't concerned what the correct name for 'it' was, what caught my attention was the likely outcome of the operation. I had never imagined myself to be likely to lose hearing in that ear, either as a result of the ailment or the treatment. At one stage I'd even hoped that there was a way the distortion could be improved. Yet instead of reading about hearing improvement I was reading about hearing loss. The papers I found strongly suggested that preservation of hearing after treatment was an exception rather than the rule. Removing the tumour either cut the nerve or damaged it to the extent that it could not function anymore. I had thought that the only problem I had was with my hearing, but I read how the close proximity of the facial nerve meant there was a significant chance that it would be damaged as well, resulting in partial facial paralysis.

I was devasted. If I thought life was difficult with damaged hearing in one ear what would it be like with no hearing in one ear? I remembered the first time I had listened to music through stereo headphones and been totally amazed at the quality of the sound. Without two ears stereo hearing is not possible; I would be deprived of one of my greatest sources of comfort and relaxation. I also knew how important first impressions are and how we all make judgements based on how people look. However much we may deny it because we think it's shallow to do so, we do. If someone dresses smartly, or trendily, or shabbily we notice and it makes a difference. If they have a lovely smile or a broken smile because one side of their face isn't working properly, we notice and it makes a difference.

I found references to other side effects that at the time I didn't understand, or try to understand. Worrying about my hearing and face kept me occupied enough. I tried to think positively; my neuroma was small, many being described were 2cm or more. Surely it would be possible to remove such a small one quite easily? I was reasonably optimistic that such devastating effects of surgery only happened when the tumour wasn't caught early enough. I reasoned that if a tumour had grown to 2cm or more then it would be much more difficult to remove. I convinced myself that as mine was small I would escape the side effects of the operation.

In retrospect that optimism was merely a coping strategy. I should have realised that the nature of the operation was such as to have serious implications whatever the size of the tumour. Maybe I should have realised, but I didn't. I just wanted something to hang some hope on, a reason to believe that I wouldn't suffer the effects of surgery I read about.

There was also a consensus that the tumours were invariably slow growing, around 2mm a year. Even so no one recommended a general wait and see policy. It seemed that the option of waiting was only for those whose general health advised against surgery, elderly patients or those with only one hearing ear.

My appointment from across the border came through along with the name of the surgeon professor I was to see. I re-checked Medline to see if he'd published anything on the subject. He had and, although it didn't add anything new to what I'd already read, I felt reassured that I was going to see someone who was indeed knowledgeable about this rare growth.

A hot sunny day in August and I was on my way to the appointment, feeling quite apprehensive but also reasonably optimistic. Everything I'd read suggested it was better to remove these things whilst they were still small. Hopefully that would mean they would be able to preserve my hearing and my normal appearance.

When I arrived at the hospital, I was first given another hearing test, this one containing an extra section of word repetition, where I had to repeat words of differing volume. After a short wait I was called in to see the Professor.

I was shown into the room and to a 'Mastermind' type chair that was in the middle of it. The Professor was sitting behind a desk working on a notebook computer while discussing something with his secretary. The nurse who had shown me in took a seat behind me. Another doctor was standing by the desk, but was apparently not actively involved with the ongoing dialogue. The discussion looked like continuing so I looked around the room and saw what looked like X ray films on the viewer.

'Are these my scans?' I asked the other doctor.

'Yes' he replied, so I got out of the chair and went over for a closer look. He came over to explain exactly what I was looking at. The scans were pictures of a succession of vertical and horizontal slices through my head. Initially it was very confusing to look at but I was slowly able to orientate myself. The tumour was very easy to see. Because I'd been injected with a dye prior to the scan it showed up as a white blob. There it was happily sitting in the auditory canal. I was surprised at how far into my head it was. Although my hearing was affected the tumour was a long way from my ear. Significantly it was still in the canal though, and hadn't started to grow out of the canal towards the brainstem. It was therefore still oblong in shape and not circular as in some of the pictures I'd seen.

With the discussion at the desk finished the Professor apologised for keeping me waiting and then asked questions about when the symptoms first began and what they were etc.. These questions seemed to take a very long time. Of course what I really wanted to know was whether I would get to keep my hearing, as I hoped. Eventually he left his desk and moved over to the scans, this time I stayed in the 'Mastermind Chair'.

'As you can see it's very close to your brainstem, maybe 3 mm away, and it could easily grow that distance in a year so it had best be removed.'

'What are the consequences of it being removed?' I asked.

'Well there are some definite and some perhaps. You will definitely lose all hearing in that ear, but I would expect to be able to preserve the facial nerve, although there are no guarantees of course. There is also a risk of not surviving the surgery, but that's now down to 1%.' He walked back to his seat behind the desk and I now felt the Mastermind Chair was a very appropriate one in which to be sitting. I had obviously been very wrong to presume that because the tumour was small it could be removed without severely detrimental side effects.

Yet again many thoughts went through my mind very quickly. Why had I not been told I could lose hearing in one ear? Why had the operation been presented to me as a straightforward one when it so obviously was not? Why was I not being offered a chance to keep my hearing when I'd read it was sometimes possible? I decided to ask:

'I've been looking up various things on Medline, and I found some people who had preserved hearing.'

'Yes, but not with the translab approach, which is the one I use. I go in through the bone behind the ear. The advantage of this is that it facilitates the preservation of the facial nerve. By using a different approach in an attempt to save hearing the facial nerve can easily be damaged and most likely the hearing will not be saved anyway. Making no attempt to save hearing maximises the chances of preserving the facial nerve.'

'I'd hoped that because mine is still small it would be possible to preserve hearing.'

'Well, although it's small it's right at the inner end of the canal. I don't normally discuss these kinds of things with patients, but as I look at the position of your tumour I wouldn't be optimistic about being able to preserve hearing. On the other hand I would be very optimistic about preserving the facial nerve. By using a different method in order to attempt to save hearing there is then more risk to the facial nerve.'

'So it's a case of aiming to save one nerve or the other, both is not possible?'

'Yes, that's more or less it. There is a trade off in that by using the translab approach the facial nerve is quite straightforward to preserve but the hearing has to be sacrificed.'

I explained that, as a musician, I valued my hearing and that I'd hoped it would be possible to preserve it.

'To be honest' he continued 'there's quite a bit of hype connected to the claims of hearing preservation. Even when it's been preserved it could have been diminished considerably, so as to be not serviceable. And even though you'll have lost hearing in one ear the distortion you complain of would go, so that would be a positive thing. But if you wanted we could try to preserve both, I did so for a gentlemen a while back. He was lucky, he got to keep both his hearing and his facial nerve.' This did not inspire me with confidence. I wanted an operation where I'd be unlucky to lose my hearing, not lucky to keep it. I'd got the message, my hearing was not realistically preservable. I decided to change track:

'It might decide to stop growing?'

'It *might*' he smiled.

'I read of a study in Denmark of a 'wait and see' policy.'

'Ah yes', he replied 'That surgeon very definitely prefers to operate when the neuroma is small. It's only really when surgery is precluded by the general health of the patient, or by their age that he advocates waiting.'

'They usually grow slowly?'

'Yes indeed they do. So if a patient is in their 70's when diagnosed their normal life expectancy is such that it's not worth operating.'

'They will most likely die before the neuroma causes serious problems?'

'Yes'.

He explained the problems I could expect as the tumour grew; initially I would suffer from facial weakness and balance problems. Then when the tumour started to compress the brain stem I would lose co-ordination. With increased brain stem compression death would eventually result.

The consultation seemed to be going nowhere. What I was being told seemed to contradict what I had read. I needed time to think. Perhaps the Professor sensed this, or perhaps the stage in the consultation had arrived where a patient is normally asking when the operation can be done and I was very definitely not.

'Well' he said, by way of a conclusion 'I don't think you're going to agree to the operation to-day so why don't we wait and scan again in 12 months time.' He mentioned another patient who had also decided on a wait and see approach, a businessman who wanted to be able to hear where voices were coming from in meetings.

'Good idea' I said, 'but isn't 12 months too long, would 6 or 9 be better?'

'No, it's fine, but if you get any new symptoms you must let us know straight away.' And he went on to explain what symptoms I should keep an eye out for, any problems with my facial muscles, or feeling. I promised I would be vigilant.

'Who knows what might happen' I said as I left 'I might be run over by a bus to-morrow, and then at least I'd die with two working ears!' They smiled and the nurse showed me out.

Sitting on the train home I went over and over the conversation in my mind. The hearing in my affected ear was quite good; the Professor himself had said so. I got the impression that it was unusual for an Acoustic Neuroma to be diagnosed with such a small amount of hearing loss. So, why should I have to sacrifice my hearing? At present the tumour wasn't doing me any great harm; so why couldn't it stay there? I needed my hearing. And I needed it not just for my work. It was difficult enough at present in crowded situations but I could imagine how that would become impossible without the ability to determine which direction a noise was coming from.

And I was concerned by the way in which the Professor had changed his mind. At the start of the consultation his attitude had been 'it's got to come out quick!', and then by the end he was happy to leave it unattended for a year. If it was OK to leave it for a year then why had he initially said that it could grow into the brainstem in that time. Either it could be left or it couldn't. How could that change? The discrepancy between what he said and what I'd read on Medline concerned me too, although not as much. It did seem possible that exaggerated claims were being made in the research articles, the 'publication bias' effect. But at the same time the claims could not be completely false, which was the Professor's implication.

The conclusion I finally came to was that the cure was worse than the disease. My only hope was that it would stop growing. Even I, with my habit of unrealistic optimism realised that was highly unlikely. Sooner or later my life was going to change; I just hoped it would be later.

However, there was something I did not know: an alternative treatment was available in a hospital less than 100 miles away. An alternative which did not involve a general anaesthetic or open surgery. An alternative which had a short term mortality rate of 0%. An alternative which had a realistic chance of hearing preservation. An alternative which could also preserve the facial nerve. I did not know because I had not been told. The ENT consultant had not told me, my GP had not told me, and the Professor had not told me. As far as I knew surgery was the only treatment available. Even though I had expressed both reluctance to undergo surgery and concern over my hearing, even though the Professor knew I was a musician who earned her living from music, I had not been told.

The alternative I had not been told about was Stereotactic Radiosurgery, which involves a single very high dose of radiation targeted at the tumour. I had not been told because the Professor does not personally believe in the treatment. Even though I was so obviously unhappy about the prospect of surgery I was not told of the existence of an alternative. The Professor allowed his own personal view and judgement to override any consideration of a 'right to know' factor. In his opinion the alternative was not a suitable treatment, therefore he denied patients knowledge of it and access to it where possible. I do not believe he had the right to do that. Of course he has the right to his opinion but surely he should have explained that another treatment was available, and then explained his reservation concerning the treatment.

I should have been told. Stereotactic Radiosurgery is not a perfect treatment, but then what is perfect? Faced with difficult choices people make decisions based on their own personality and circumstances. When asked to choose between conventional surgery and radiosurgery many people choose conventional surgery, others choose radiosurgery. The important thing is that the patient has made an informed choice. People are more than the sum of their constituent cells and however talented a surgeon may be he cannot make decisions of that nature on behalf of the patient. He can advise and express opinions but the ultimate decision should be the patient's, after all they are the one who are going to have to live with the results of that decision. I therefore think that the Professor should have had more faith in his treatment and told me of the alternative. By not doing so he weakened his own case rather than strengthened it.

Furthermore the Professor had refused to accept the limitations of his own personal judgement. Despite his own conviction not all the medical profession actually agree with him. An article advocating the use of Stereotactic Radiosurgery was to appear in the British Medical Journal within a few months. But on that train journey home I was completely unaware of its existence and I should not have been. I felt that my only chance of retaining my hearing was the medical equivalent of winning the lottery.

Chapter Three

Home - The World – and Back

1. Home!

The next few months were difficult and stressful. On that journey home I never wondered what the reaction of people would be, but I must have had a subconscious idea of what I would have liked it to be as over the following weeks I frequently found myself feeling confused and hurt during conversations with others.

Most people seemed to be of the opinion that if the tumour was going to have to be removed eventually it was better to do it sooner rather than later. This reaction took the form of 'Once the operation's over with you can start to get on with your life again, get used to one-sided deafness, put it all behind you.' My response was I'd rather preserve my bilateral hearing as long as possible, that I doubted whether I was capable of adjusting to life with hearing in only one ear. I got the impression that even though I was a musician, most people did not view the lack of hearing in one ear as a serious problem. I found this very puzzling as I could see very many problems. I had already begun to avoid going to live concerts but I was still able to enjoy listening to music at home by using headphones. If I lost hearing in one ear then this would become impossible, effectively meaning that listening to music would no longer be possible. Stress is something we have to learn how to control, to avoid an excess of. Listening to music is my way of dealing with stress so to be deprived of that would be extremely difficult. I was not at all sure how unilateral hearing would affect my ability to teach the piano, but I thought it very likely I would simply not be able to hear enough detail to do my job properly.

I could see how social events and work meetings would become so difficult that some would be impossible. This difficulty would extend to everyday activities such as going for a drink or having a meal with a few friends and not be confined to major events such as weddings. When I later met people who had lost hearing in one ear this view was confirmed; they said crowded events were so difficult and so tiring that it was better not to attend.

Although attention tended to focus on hearing, as deafness in one ear was a certainty, I was also genuinely concerned that I may not survive the operation, or that I might sustain facial nerve damage as well. Again, other people did not seem to share my concerns.

People viewed the 1% mortality rate as a negligible risk, but I did not think so. If someone was placed in a room with 100 revolvers, only one of which was loaded, would they willingly pick one up at random and fire it at their head? Obviously not. If the choice became 'Either pick up one of those or you're going to be shot anyway' then most people would take the risk. But I was not in that situation. At that time the tumour was not in any way threatening my life, so why should I take such a risk to have it removed?

People attempted to re-assure me that if I did suffer facial nerve damage those close to me would not view me any differently, they would get used to the way I looked. However, my concern was not about the reaction of those who knew me well, but of those who did not. I would not spend all of my time with those close to me and society reacts to the way people look. However much we may complain about our beauty culture and obsession with appearances, it exists. In magazines we see photographs of beautiful young men, women, children and babies being used to promote the sale of various products. It is difficult enough for those of us who have the normal assortment of overlarge tummies, odd shaped noses, straggly hair etc.. How much more difficult must it be for those who have suffered some actual disfigurement. Even very young children have been shown to react more favourably to other children who are considered attractive. I knew that a half paralysed or half-droopy face would not receive a favourable reaction. Going out would be difficult, and although I had no wish to become a recluse maybe that would be less painful than people's reactions to my new features. When I later met patients whose facial nerve had been damaged I realised my fears were justified.

Along with this 'better to get it over with' reaction tended to go the 'expert theory', which went along the lines of: 'These people know what they're doing. It's amazing what they can do these days. I'm sure it will be OK.' Whilst I do have a genuine respect for the skills of medical people my reaction to the expert theory was to ask why, if they were so skilled, wasn't it possible to remove the 'thing in my head' without sacrificing my hearing and running so many other serious risks?

As time went on I began to feel increasingly isolated. I'm sure that no one intended anything other than support and friendly advice in their comments, but my confused and stressed mind didn't receive them happily. 'At least you'll still have hearing in the other ear'; 'I wouldn't back a horse at 100 to one'; 'things will get back to normal once you've had the operation'; are but a few. All were said in an attempt to help, but they didn't. I found that there were very, very few people I could actually talk to; counting them on one hand would still have left most fingers spare. It seemed that the ability to listen and to make comments that would not in some way be upsetting was a rare ability indeed. So I began to not talk about the thing in my head. Because conversations were so frequently upsetting I stopped mentioning it, and as the symptoms began to worsen so my sense of isolation increased. I began to feel a constant pressure on the affected side and to suffer from increasingly frequent and severe headaches. However, I felt I couldn't really say anything as to do so invoked the 'maybe it's time to get it treated' response. Even the word 'treated' invoked a negative response in me. In my view surgery was not a treatment; treatments were supposed to make you better not worse.

I realised people didn't understand just how serious the situation was as they spoke of me being 'cured' and 'getting better'. Even the best result of surgical removal was not what I viewed as a cure, but my attempts to explain the seriousness of the situation were only met by attempts at reassurance, which I found upsetting, so I stopped trying. I also felt hurt. I am not and never have been a person who moans about their health, or assumes every ache and pain means imminent death. That should have been sufficient reason in itself to convince others of the seriousness of the situation, but it wasn't.

What I needed to hear, but only very occasionally did hear, was that it was OK to be worried, that it wasn't just a bad cold I was suffering from, that it was serious. Only when I thought that the nature of the problem was understood was it possible to discuss ways forward.

Looking back I wonder if I would have dealt with myself in the same way. If it had been a friend diagnosed and not me would I have reacted any differently? Of course I like to think that if the situation had been reversed I would have been one of the very few people who actually understood and was easy to talk to about it, but in reality who knows? Perhaps, for most people, it is only by going through an experience that the ability to help and understand others is gained. I certainly notice now that if a friend is in a seemingly impossible situation from which there is no way out my response is 'That's awful, you must feel really bad', and discuss the options. I certainly now would not attempt to be reassuring and say 'I'm sure it will turn out fine' as I know just how unhelpful, and hurtful, such false reassurances are.

At times my confidence in my own interpretation of the situation wavered and I thought that so many people could not be mistaken; therefore I must be. The seriousness of the situation was understood and I was simply making too much of it. As a child I'm sure that words along the lines of 'Don't make a fuss, just get on with it' had been said to me many times with justification. Young children make a huge fuss at the slightest accident so they are encouraged to make less fuss, making a fuss is babyish. As adults, we all have met people who moan constantly about their health even though their health is no worse than that of the rest of us. Although I doubt many of us actually say it, we have all at some stage probably thought something like 'Why don't they just shut up and get on with it.' Was I now being classed with those people? Had I just become a 'whinger'? Was I reacting unreasonably? Was the operation merely a routine kind of thing no worse than having an appendix removed? Was I being completely unreasonable and totally over-reacting? Should I therefore just 'shut up and get on with it'?

As well as those who constantly moan, we have also all met people who forever try to tell others how to do their job, or those who believe they are an authority on every subject mentioned. Such people are not popular and are considered arrogant. Being arrogant is frowned upon. So whenever someone said to me 'These people are experts, they know what is best,' instead of it reassuring me I questioned my own questioning of them. How could I possibly not take the advice of the experts? This merely served to confuse me considerably as I did not gain any increase in trust, I just felt guilty for not trusting.

My GP, who initially had been so helpful, was very definitely in the 'better to get it over with' group. He could see no benefit at all in waiting and probably couldn't see exactly what I was waiting for. Could I see what I was waiting for? Not exactly, no. I suppose I had a very strong feeling that there just had to be a less destructive treatment somewhere it was just a case of finding it. It was obvious that if there was an alternative treatment no-one, including the medics, was going to find it for me, I just had to start looking myself.

2. The World.

Those of you who can remember it will be aware of the phenomenal growth of the world wide web (www) in the late 1990's. Initially very few people had internet access at home and the early dial up connections were extremely slow and somewhat unreliable. But I was lucky in having access through the University, and I was about to spend considerable amounts of time 'talking' to people thousands of miles away. What is striking is how I found more information about the UK from people in America than I did from anyone in the UK. Striking and depressing.

First of all I found the address of the Acoustic Neuroma Association in America and they sent me lots of information, together with the address of the British Acoustic Neuroma Association. Given the acknowledged importance of patient support groups why had nobody here told me of their existence? I wondered why it was not common practice to inform patients of relevant support groups, particularly when the ailment is not a common condition. I had met no one that had an Acoustic Neuroma and met no one who knew anyone who had one.

The information sent by the Neuroma Associations included practical details on the operational procedure itself. I learned that it was a long operation, anywhere between 6 and 16 hours. A few days had to be spent in intensive care afterwards, which was followed by at least a week on the ward.

Driving was prohibited for around 6 weeks. Patients could expect to be off work for that time at the very least and more likely 6 months. As a mother of 2 young children I knew that to be 'off work' was not possible. As soon as I returned home I would be expected to read stories, play games and find lost toys. Later when I met, or wrote to, people who had undergone the operation I was to learn just how much the operation could change working life. Many had to change to part-time work and some had given up work completely. There just had to be an alternative way.

I continued my internet search and finally one day read of an alternative treatment to surgery: Gamma Knife. As I delved I discovered more. The first Gamma Knife machine had been built in 1968 in Stockholm at the Karolinska Institute. Professor Leksell, head of the team, called the new technique 'stereotactic radiosurgery'. 'Stereotactic' in reference to the guiding devices used to pinpoint the tumour and 'radiosurgery' as it's surgery which uses radiation not a knife. The patient is fitted, by means of screws, with a head frame and onto the frame is fitted a helmet which contains many small holes. The radiation passes through the holes and is focussed on the tumour. As well as being used to treat Acoustic Neuromas, the technique is also used to treat other benign brain tumours and arteriovenous malformations (AVMs).

The claims made about the success of the treatment on the hospital websites looked very good: an impressive percentage of patients retained their pre-treatment hearing levels; the risk of facial nerve damage was reduced; there were no reported deaths as a result of treatment; the procedure could be performed without the need for a general anaesthetic so the length of hospital stay was approximately a mere 48 hours. The contrast between Gamma Knife and conventional surgery was stark. Conventional surgery was a risky procedure involving a length hospital stay; Gamma Knife a minimally invasive 2 night stay. But were these website claims exaggerated or realistic? I needed to find what was in the published medical research literature.

So it was back to Medline, this time looking up Stereotactic Radiosurgery. In particular, I was looking for a study comparing conventional surgery with Gamma Knife treatment.

The classic experimental design for a study comparing two different treatments is a Randomised Controlled Trial (RCT). Here patients are given information on the purpose of the study, invited to participate and if they agree are randomly assigned to different treatment groups. If it's a drug treatment the treating physician does not know which group the patient has been allocated to, and the patient does not know which group they have been allocated to. Furthermore, when the results are being analysed the researchers don't know which group is which; it is only at the very end that this information is given. There can be ethical problems with this design though; in the treatment of Acoustic Neuroma would it be ethical to assign patients to either surgery or radiosurgery purely at random? I think not. This does not mean it is impossible to conduct a valid comparison, just that a different design is needed and that care must be taken to match the two groups of patients as closely as possible. Despite that some critics will still argue that the only way to make a true comparison is through a Randomised Controlled Trial.

During my search, I was surprised by how vague some of the measures used in the publications were. For example, some authors claimed that 'useful hearing' was preserved in percentage of their patients. But the description 'useful hearing' actually means very little as it is simply too vague. It may be useful to have sufficient hearing on the affected side to be able to hear an approaching lorry when crossing the road, but such hearing may be useless in terms of understanding speech. Of more value is a description such as 'pre-treatment' hearing levels were maintained, thereby indicating the impact of the procedure on hearing levels.

However, after spending many days searching it became apparent that the claims made by the hospitals on their web sites were endorsed by the literature. In particular the Pittsburgh Medical Center, USA, had published good results and had also published the results of a study which compared conventional surgery with radiosurgery. The Gamma Knife treatment technique looked good, so why wasn't it done here in the UK, or was it? I faxed, e-mailed and wrote letters to hospitals in America and Sweden and from them discovered that there indeed was a Gamma Knife machine in the UK; the fourth machine ever to be built in the 1980's.

Reassured that the Gamma Knife treatment would presumably be available if that was the way I decided to go I set about finding as much as I could about it, and it was during my renewed search on the internet I discovered e-mail discussion groups.

From the Acoustic Neuroma Associations, the email discussion group and Web Sites I discovered powerful arguments for and against both surgery and

Gamma Knife. I realised that there were even more side effects of surgery than I had been told about. Headaches may actually worsen after surgery or even appear for the first time; problems with eyes in terms of 'dry eye' or non-functioning eyelids were frequently mentioned. I read of complications such as hydrocephalus, (the treatment for which was to insert a tube to drain away excess fluid from around the brain) and meningitis. The list of complications just seemed to grow and grow! I also learned that removing the tumour surgically did not mean it would not grow again, a possibility that had not been mentioned to me.

After lurking in the background for awhile I decided to put some direct questions to the discussion group, requesting opinions on the relative merits of surgery and radiosurgery. The replies confirmed my suspicions; there was a huge medical disagreement about the treatment of Acoustic Neuroma. Surgeons wanted to cut; radiosurgeons couldn't see the point in cutting when it was possible to treat without. The main arguments against Gamma Knife all seemed to be based on the long-term prognosis, and in this long-term argument the proponents of surgery had a very powerful weapon – cancer. Acoustic Neuromas are almost invariably benign; although they grow they remain encapsulated and do not spread to other parts of the body. The pro-surgery lobby stated that by using radiation on a benign tumour there was a likelihood of it turning malignant, and of course malignant tumours are something we all want to avoid.

Another argument against the Gamma Knife surfaced: that the tumour was more likely to grow again following radiosurgery than microsurgery and if it did the effects of the radiation on the tumour would make surgery more difficult. It was claimed that the radiation melted the tumour and nerves together making it almost impossible to remove the tumour without nerve damage.

Of course the Gamma Knife proponents had answers for their critics stating that patients in Sweden had been treated using the Gamma Knife since the late 1960's and there was no evidence of it causing malignancy. On the question as to whether radiosurgery made future surgery more difficult there was further disagreement; some said 'yes', some said 'no'. And it was complicated by some surgeons offering the opinion that if a tumour needed to be operated on after re-growth following conventional surgery it was also considerably more difficult.

There was apparently no one answer. If I opted for surgery I ran very real risks and would certainly lose hearing in my right ear. If I opted for radiosurgery I could still gradually lose hearing in one ear and the risk of facial nerve damage, although less, was still there. A decision based on short term outcome was an easy one to make. Conventional surgery was a much more invasive, riskier and complicated option; Gamma Knife was the obvious choice. The huge question mark hung over the long-term risks. Once surgery was done it was done. If I survived the operation and the time in intensive care then the risks would be over provided it didn't grow again. Whereas, if the proponents of surgery were to be believed, the risk of death from Gamma Knife treatment was just delayed by 10 years or more. After reading the heart-rending messages sent by people to the brain tumour group I knew that it would be an extremely painful and distressing death. On the other hand if I didn't survive conventional surgery I would presumably know nothing about it. It was an impossible decision to make.

3. Home Again.

To decide between the two treatment options I needed to discuss them with people who had more medical knowledge than me. Armed with the information I had found it was time to tackle the medical people locally to see what their opinion was.

My first contact was my GP and I told him what I'd found on the internet. He was unimpressed. His opinion was that 'average', 'normal' patients would not join discussion groups or Acoustic Neuroma Associations, so they did not represent a fair sample of patients. Whilst I accepted that point, as I was myself already aware that only people with problems would join the group, he seemed to dismiss all information obtained from those sources purely on those grounds. I could not agree with that attitude as I could see how I could easily become one of those patients. These people were not inventing their problems; they were real and were in accordance with what I had read in the published literature.

The fact that the information had originated from America didn't help either. My GP's opinion was that a treatment other than surgery would be favoured in the US as it would be cheaper etc.. His conclusion was that if the treatment were a viable one the Professor would have mentioned it to me. Back again to the 'expert' theory. These people, among them the Professor, are experts and I was not, so I should not question their decision. I was definitely made to feel that I was being arrogant by being so persistent in my questions. The GP seemed to think I was under the delusion I knew better than the Professor. It was very upsetting to feel I was being looked on in that way. I did not consider that I knew more, I was simply of the view that a person whose specialisation was in one area would perhaps not be very favourable to other treatment options. To me it was an issue of human nature, an issue my GP did not consider.

Conversations with the ENT consultant did not improve things. His opinion was the same: if the Gamma Knife treatment were a successful treatment the Professor would have mentioned it. So I sent him the Pittsburgh article comparing surgery and radiosurgery treatment outcomes. The claims made in the article are impressive: radiosurgery was found to be more effective in preserving hearing; in preserving normal facial nerve function; patients returned to being able to look after themselves much sooner, and complications following treatment were less. However, this article was criticised as it did not use randomised techniques, the patients themselves chose whether to have surgery or radiosurgery. As I mentioned earlier I find this criticism extraordinary; surely it would be unethical to NOT let the patient make such an important decision. My attempts to persuade the consultant that because the groups had been matched according to tumour size etc. the results were still valid failed completely. He continued to maintain that the Professor was the expert and if the treatment were worth doing he would have suggested it.

By now I was in a pretty poor and very confused state. I did not know which treatment was the best. Although not a perfect treatment radiosurgery definitely seemed to offer the better hope of a successful outcome. My only concern, albeit a major concern, was the alleged risk of incurring malignancy. I knew that the chance of not surviving surgery was 1%, what I wanted to quantify was the chance of developing a malignant tumour. I needed to find a piece of long term research. But it was not there. Even though the Gamma Knife treatment had been available for so many years I could find nothing that had followed patients for more than 4 or 5 years. I thought that given the huge controversy surrounding treatment alternatives one of the patient groups, either the British or American Acoustic Neuroma Associations, or perhaps both, would have taken responsibility for the research, but they had not.

At around the same time a friend showed me an article about Acoustic Neuroma treatment from a recent issue of The British Medical Journal and it predicted that radiosurgery would become the standard treatment for a small Acoustic Neuroma. As the article had been co-written by a surgeon I felt it carried some weight.

I found myself increasingly wishing that I could go somewhere which carried out both procedures, so they could look at my tumour and explain the pros and cons of each treatment in my individual case. Although a very sensible wish it was apparently unattainable. By now I realised that the Professor fell into the 'surgery is best in all cases' camp and so I expected no help from him. But what about the ENT department of my own local hospital? They could not carry out any treatment at all, neither surgery nor radiosurgery, so they had nothing to gain by preferring one treatment to another. I thought they should have been aware of the different treatment options and been able to offer unbiased advice. However the attitude of the department was very much to carry on doing things as they always had done, why change? They had always recommended neurosurgery and had apparently never questioned whether it was the best, or only, treatment.

The time for my next scan was approaching and therefore if the tumour had grown so was decision time. I was aware of a great deal of pressure to have surgery and frequently felt it to be the best option. In trying to make my decision I looked for more research evidence, which was not there. My response to that was to believe that if I looked harder, delved deeper, then I would find the necessary research results somewhere.

Eventually a friend helped me to realise that the reason I could not find the results was simply because they were not there; however hard I looked I would not find them.

But I was concentrating so hard on finding facts that I totally neglected to consider why I was reacting in the way I was to the facts I had. I should have tried harder to separate fact from feeling rather than trying to find enough facts to silence any feelings. No treatment actually 'felt' to be the best treatment overall, but I frequently felt that surgery was the most appropriate option. What I was unaware of, and didn't really consider, was where the feeling that surgery was the most appropriate was coming from. Now, with the benefit of hindsight, (that greatest asset of all!) I can understand that the feeling that surgery was better was largely caused by external forces which were masquerading as internal.

I appreciate now that we are all under tremendous pressure to conform to what is expected of us and it is not easy to withstand that pressure. Furthermore, we are brought up to believe that in many areas someone else will 'know what's best'; the smooth running of our society depends on it. We cannot all be experts on every topic which affects our lives.

By having surgery I would be deferring to the experts, the higher authority, and thereby absolving myself of the decision-making responsibility. If I had surgery and it went wrong everyone would say 'You were very unlucky but you weren't to know, you made the right decision at the time'. They would be sympathetic and make all the right noises. I would not be to blame.

On the other hand if I had radiosurgery and that went wrong people would say 'Perhaps surgery would have been better after all, we did try to tell you at the time'. In addition, it would be my own fault; I would be to blame. I would be seen to have refused to listen to all the 'experts'. 'Well she got what she deserved, should have listened to the experts' would be a likely response.

I therefore experienced a huge inner conflict; the external pressures combined to make surgery *feel* as if it were the best option, yet when I looked at the evidence concerning both treatments I could see that was not necessarily the case. Unfortunately I could not see what actually was the case. When I felt that surgery was the best option even though I could see that it wasn't I interpreted that as meaning that I needed more information. Maybe I did, maybe if I had found just one good piece of longitudinal research it would have silenced the voices. But also, maybe if I had better understood my own reactions the conflicting voices would have been silenced with the information I had.

If one treatment had indeed been the perfect treatment I would not have experienced such a dilemma. But life is full of grey, shady areas of decision making and in negotiating such areas we need to be fully aware of the nature of the influences which bear upon us; something I very definitely was not. My insight into my own thought processes and feelings was at the time only marginally greater than zero. I could not get past a vague awareness that in some weird way having surgery would be an easy way out. But I also wondered if it was my body trying to tell me something. Was it actually the wisest course of action to take? Did surgery feel right because it was right?

Chapter Four

Gamma Knife

The day before my then husband's birthday I had a very frustrating trip to England for the follow up scan. I myself had no idea whether the tumour had grown or not. As far as I could tell my hearing was the same and my facial nerve was not affected. However, I was also becoming increasingly aware of pressure on the affected side. It was as if I could feel something pressing on the bone behind my ear from the inside, creating a constant dull ache. It was not something which was particularly painful, rather a dull ache which was always there. But did it mean that the tumour was growing? I needed to have a scan to find out.

The train journey took a long three hours and on the way I felt quite apprehensive as to what the scan would show. The contrast in my attitude to the previous scan did not escape my attention. Before I had only been concerned about the actual procedure, in that instance ignorance had, well and truly, been bliss. But now I was not concerned about the procedure, but I was extremely concerned about the result. I was hoping so much that the tumour would not have grown but at the same time was very much aware that my symptoms were getting worse, and how could they get worse unless the tumour was growing?

Unlike my local hospital, which only had the articulated lorry version of the scanner, the large city hospital had a permanent one. The scanner itself was much more user friendly; I could listen to music, there was a light inside and I was given a panic button to hold. The nurse explained that if at any stage I wanted to come out of the machine I just had to press the button and they would come and get me. It's odd how such a simple little thing can make such a big difference. Simply *knowing* that I could press the button was in itself very re-assuring and made me feel much happier.

I explained to the nurse that I knew I had a tumour and was anxious to know whether or not it had grown since my last scan. She explained something about only doctors being able to give out information. So I asked if she could simply tell me whether or not it was still in the auditory canal. She didn't respond and slid me into the machine. This time I knew what to expect and so did not open my eyes at all. The music was playing but when the scanner was working it was again very noisy, so noisy that I simply could not hear the music at all. However, I could hear it during the pauses in the procedure and did find it relaxing.

In due course the scanner became silent and I felt the table sliding me back out into the world again. I asked the nurse if the tumour was still in the auditory canal and she replied that she would see if there was a doctor available. So I returned to the changing room and replaced the gown with my own clothes, jewellery was retrieved from the locker and I waited by the door through which the medical people disappeared. No-one seemed to be either coming in or going out. I was at a complete loss as to what to do. I waited and waited but nothing happened so I decided to go and speak to the receptionist. I told her what the nurse had said and she asked me to wait while she went to check. Unfortunately, she was quickly back with the news that there was no doctor available, I would received a letter in due course.

As I left the hospital I felt quite numb initially and then rather annoyed. This I could do without. It was stressful enough having the thing in my head without people acting in ways which were guaranteed to increase the stress. I could understand why an appointment had to be made to give an initial diagnosis but why could somebody not have found 1 minute to speak to me? It was not as if the scanner was operated single handedly? And unlike blood and tissue samples which have to be sent for analysis the scan of my head was on the computer screen during the procedure. All I wanted to know was whether the tumour was still in the auditory canal and I had to leave the hospital without that knowledge.

I walked into the city centre and tried to concentrate on what to buy as a birthday present. But I couldn't. I wandered into shop after shop but found that my thoughts kept returning to 'has it grown, when will I get a letter, what will I do if it has grown, etc. etc.'. Birthday presents seemed to not be sufficiently compelling to distract me from those thoughts. Eventually I wandered into Marks and Spencer and bought a shirt. A very safe shirt in a very safe colour; totally unlike the ones I knew I should have been looking at, but to choose one of those would have required concentration, and I couldn't concentrate.

If chaos theory states that the flap of a butterfly's wings in India can cause a hurricane on the other side of the world then it will come as no surprise that the lack of information given after the scan resulted in a boring birthday present!

Without knowing whether the tumour had grown or not I had to consider the possibility that it had and that meant considering which treatment to have. I knew that the Professor would urge me to have surgery; I had to find out more about the only alternative I knew of: Gamma Knife.

I had become so accustomed to a lack of home grown information that it didn't strike me as particularly strange that a contact in America gave me the phone number of the appropriate person. I had a name and a number but I was still extremely apprehensive about phoning. The contact I'd had with medical people so far had been such a negative experience; would new people be any different? However, I knew that the logical course of action was to obtain an appointment to see the Gamma Knife people, so however unpleasant I found the prospect there was no alternative but to phone. No-one was going to do so on my behalf, I just had to get on and do it.

I was very worried about what the reaction of the hospital would be to me, a mere patient, phoning. I considered it a real possibility that they would actually refuse to speak to me, insisting that I be referred by my local hospital, which I knew would not happen. I knew the ENT consultant did not consider Gamma Knife to be a valid treatment and suspected he would actually refuse to refer me. If that happened what were my options? Would I even have any options? I felt completely powerless. Even though it was my head and my health which were at stake I knew that the power lay with others.

I've always found that the best time to make a difficult phone call is first thing in the morning. Any later and it becomes all too easy to put it off until another day! At least I had a name to ask for. That was the only positive thing I could think of as I phoned – the receptionist wouldn't ask awkward questions!

Still, I was shaking when I phoned. I was quickly put through to the correct person and I explained my situation. Immediately my apprehension vanished, the person I spoke to was understanding and sympathetic to. She agreed that the best thing would be for me to have a consultation as soon as possible. When explaining that I would need to be referred by someone her manner was again supportive, apologising for it being a necessary piece of red tape. Although an unusual situation as most referrals are made by consultants, she was happy for my GP to write the letter. We arranged for my scans, hearing test results etc. to be copied and sent on. As I put the phone down I simply felt numb, I couldn't believe it, I had, for the first time spoken to a medical person who seemed to be a real person and who in return treated me as if I too were a real person. For the first time I felt as if my wishes were being taken into consideration, that it was only natural and correct that I should have a say in what treatment I had.

The appointment came through within a few weeks and then it was an even longer train journey into England. The day was bitterly cold and the train journey was very long, cold and uncomfortable. Thankfully once there the hospital waiting area was very warm. In due course I was shown into a consulting room and this time there were no other staff present. As usual I had to explain the progression of my symptoms.

'Looking at your hearing tests your hearing is very good, comparatively.' commented the consultant.

'I know', I replied 'that's why I'm so reluctant to lose it in the operation!'

'Understandably. It could be that the tumour is actually growing on the vestibular portion of the nerve, causing most damage to that. Have you had a vestibular function test?'

'No, just hearing tests.'

'Well, I think we should get one organised, I'm sure that your local hospital will be able to carry one out.'
He then put my most recent scan onto the X ray viewer. I anxiously got up to have a closer look as I still hadn't heard whether it had grown or not. The verdict was immediately apparent - the tumour had definitely grown. On the first scan it was contained completely within the auditory canal, now it had grown out of the canal and was beginning to form a circle about 2mm in diameter.

I asked if the original scans had been sent as well.

'No, apparently not.' he replied. 'Have they calculated the volume of the tumour?'

I replied that as far as I knew they had not, and explained what the tumour looked like on the first scan.

'Without a volume calculation it's difficult to assess its actual rate of growth, we always do them for that reason. But looking at your tumour there is absolutely no rush to do anything right now. I would suggest re-scanning in a year and then making a decision.'

I asked him about hearing preservation and likely facial nerve damage. His replies confirmed what I had read in the literature; that he could not guarantee to preserve hearing, but that if it did fade it would do so gradually, which I knew would be easier to cope with. He was equally honest with regard to possible facial nerve damage.

I then asked if it was indeed more difficult to operate should the tumour begin to grow after GK treatment.

'There is no reason why the GK treatment cannot be carried out again – until someone reaches their maximum radiation dose that is. There's a lot of discussion about the optimum dose at present. I think that perhaps Stockholm have gone too low now and that some tumours may continue to grow. On the other hand the early doses given were too high so there was damage to hearing and facial nerves.'

We chatted in general about the treatment at Pittsburgh and Stockholm and it was reassuring to be able to discuss what I had read. Finally, I felt that I was being treated as someone who had a worthwhile contribution to make to the treatment decision, and my wish to preserve my hearing was respected and acknowledged.

When the allotted consultation time was over I was asked if I wished to have a further consultation. I replied that I didn't, that I was happy to wait and have another scan the following February.

For the first time since I'd been referred I left a consultation feeling reasonably content. I still wished that the tumour would go away and I still did not want to have any treatment at all. But what I was happy about was that the consultant had been honest with me and I felt confident that he would not try to persuade me to have treatment before it was necessary. He also had not tried to hide any of the downsides of the treatment. So although not a perfect treatment, and still not what I would have previously regarded as a treatment, I thought that it was a less destructive option. I was still clinging onto my favourite option however – that in a year's time the tumour would not have grown and I could delay action even longer.

The journey home was equally long and uncomfortable and I was extremely tired as the day had begun at 5 am. However, at least by now the trains had warmed up! And, having had a proper conversation about possible treatment I was reasonably content. So rather than fretting and worrying I spent the journey home wondering why nice trains only seem to run north – south, and whether that's the same in other countries too!

Chapter Five

To Go Where Only Fools Dare To Tread?

It was a couple of weeks later that I finally heard from the Professor. I received a letter stating that the tumour was still small, so he suggested having a scan and consultation later in the year. It felt like I was reading the score when I'd already watched the match, so the letter was filed away and I tried to forget about surgery and Gamma Knife – and the tumour itself. The summer drifted by, my hearing remained the same, the tinnitus remained the same, and the feeling of pressure inside my head remained the same. Or was that getting worse and I just wasn't aware of it?

However, my attempts to behave like an ostrich were well and truly scuppered when I received a letter from the ENT consultant at my local hospital. He had received a phone call from the Professor who was very concerned at my considering Gamma Knife as a treatment. I was strongly urged to keep the appointment later in the year in order that the issue could be discussed. My instinctive reaction was to definitely **not** keep the appointment. I knew that both the ENT consultant and the Professor were not in favour of the treatment; therefore I assumed that any consultation would be an attempt to dissuade me. Half of me simply couldn't be bothered; I just didn't want the hassle and almost inevitable emotional upset of that meeting.

But the other half of me considered that I should attend. If I had indeed got my facts right there would be nothing new that the Professor could say. Friends and family very much considered that I should go, that he should be given the opportunity to state his case and explain why he didn't approve of Gamma Knife treatment. So I replied that I would keep the appointment and I would listen to what the Professor had to say. After behaving like an ostrich over the summer it was back to reality. I felt very apprehensive about the forthcoming consultation. At times it seemed as if my permanent mental state was one of apprehension, and it seemed that way because that's the way it was.

At least this time I knew I would get to know the result of the scan the same day as I was scheduled to have the scan late morning and see the Professor early afternoon.

By now I was used to the MRI procedure and although not a pleasant experience I had learned the best way for me to deal with it. I took the Dudley Moore piano CD with me again and kept my eyes closed for the duration of the scan. An unfortunate side effect is that I still can't listen to the CD without thinking I'm in the machine! A shame, because there's some lovely music on it.

A mere 10 minutes after the scan I was given an envelope to take with me to the consultation. For some reason it never entered my head to look at the contents of the envelope for a sneak preview. I handed in the envelope and was summoned for a hearing test before the actual consultation. As before the Professor was not alone, his secretary sat to one side of him and a nurse sat quietly at the back of the room. As I entered the room I looked around to see if my scans were on the X Ray viewer, they were not. Once more I had to sit in the Mastermind chair in the middle of the room.

'Well,' said the Professor as I sat down 'your tumour hasn't changed, it's exactly the same as it was in February.' I felt enormous relief, and disbelief.

'Could I see it?' I asked. He looked surprised but put the scan on the viewer for me to see. It could have been the same scan as the one I looked at in February. No change at all.

'I understand that you're considering Stereotactic Radiation.' Well, at least he got straight to the point. 'It's no wonder cure you know. You could still lose your hearing after it, and there's more of a risk to the facial nerve as I'm almost certain I could preserve it in an operation.'

'I know it's not guaranteed' I replied, 'but at least if my hearing does go it will happen gradually, which would be easier to cope with than a sudden overnight loss. And I'm aware that there's a risk to the facial nerve as well.'

'There's also the risk of malignancy,' he continued. It seemed as if his first statement hadn't had the desired effect so he continued along lines which were guaranteed to have an effect. He claimed that people who had received radiosurgery were now being found to have malignant tumours as a result. My first reaction was to wonder why I had found no reference to it in the medical literature. I needed more information.

'Where has it been happening?' I asked, thinking that I would need to know that in order to ascertain whether or not it was true.

'Well in Denmark they're turning up in droves after being treated in Stockholm. And they've had one or two cases in Pittsburgh as well.' For some reason I noticed his secretary, who although silent had a 'well that's put her in her place' expression on her face.

The Professor continued by saying that he didn't believe in radiosurgery treatment and if I was unwise enough to want to go ahead with it he would not refer me. He then continued to express his conviction that he could save the facial nerve, which was responded to with my desire to keep my hearing. I felt that he was definitely trying to persuade me to have surgery. He tried to reassure me that although I would lose my hearing in the affected ear the distortion in my ear would go too. He also said that a lot of patients stated that they could actually hear better following the operation. And of course he was very confident about preserving my facial nerve.

I suddenly became very tired and began to wonder when the next train was. The consultation was going nowhere except round in circles. The Professor seemed very happy to continue talking about surgery and what it could achieve but I'd had enough, I wanted to go home.

'Well, as it hasn't grown,' I began by way of concluding the consultation 'I'd still like to do nothing, because I think that at the present time any treatment would actually make me feel worse.'

He looked relieved. 'I think you're right, it would. Your tumour's still small so we could scan again in a year's time.'

'Fine, maybe I'll get lucky – maybe it will stop growing completely!'

I left the consultation feeling like a huge ordeal had been managed successfully. But why was it an ordeal?

Why was it so difficult to discuss the treatment options? Why did I feel as if I was going into some sort of battle? Why did I feel threatened rather than supported? Probably because it wasn't an actual discussion. I knew what the Professor wanted me to do and I knew what he thought of me for considering alternatives. But why should that be upsetting? It's OK for people to disagree isn't it? Well no, with some people the choice is presented as being between 'their way and the wrong way'. Perhaps not everyone would find that situation upsetting; in fact I can think of a few people who would positively relish it. But I don't remember ever being a 'Rebel Without a Cause' character or even a 'Rebel With a Cause'! I don't like confrontation. So what was someone like me doing disagreeing with an eminent surgeon? Trying to preserve my hearing, perhaps my face, maybe even my life. I knew that the Professor was confident about the operation, but I also knew that things can go wrong and that the only way to absolutely guarantee that the operation would not go wrong was to not have it.

Many months later I heard of someone who underwent the identical operation to remove a tumour of a similar size to my own. He too had been assured that surgery was the best alternative and although vaguely aware of alternatives trusted the judgement of the surgeon. Like the Professor his surgeon had been extremely confident about preserving the facial nerve. But the reality was totally different. When he recovered from the operation he was told that his facial nerve had been cut resulting in total facial paralysis on the affected side. He then contracted meningitis and was in hospital for a total of 4 weeks. He contacted me 12 weeks later and was having eye problems because one eye was so dry, and on top of everything he couldn't walk in a straight line. He managed to write all of that without any trace of bitterness. I doubt very much I could have done the same. But it was a strange feeling reading his story – that so, so easily could have been me.

And some years later I met a lady who'd had a tumour the same size as mine which the Professor had operated on to remove. He'd given her the identical reassurances he gave me, but it hadn't worked out as planned; the facial nerve was damaged and she only had half a smile.

Those are just two of the many examples of people I subsequently met where things had not gone as planned. For so many people things seemed to go wrong.

Which has made me wonder whether we have come to expect too much of medicine, and my personal opinion is that we have. In particular, we have become blasé about surgical procedures and now view them as routine and almost without risk. But there always is a risk, there's the risk of the anaesthetic and a risk that the procedure will go wrong. We forget that in our desire to alleviate worry and stress, but sometimes it is good to be worried, worry makes us cautious and caution is essential for self preservation. To every individual and their family each procedure carries a risk and however unpleasant it is to do so we need to remember that fact. Hiding behind the reassurance of 'It's amazing what they can do these days' will ultimately not be productive. A small percentage of surgical procedures will always go wrong. The percentage may well be small, and hopefully will continue to get smaller, but will always be there. We don't want to, but we need to retain a respect for surgery, we need to be worried.

However skilled the team are, however sophisticated the equipment is there can never be any guarantees. For the family of the 1% of people who do not survive Acoustic Neuroma surgery it is absolutely no consolation to know that 99% do survive, that they were just unlucky. How could that be any consolation when they have lost a person they love and treasure. The only consolation would be to know that there had been no alternative, that unless the operation had been carried out the patient would have died or led an intolerable life.

Amazingly, the idea that surgery can be a routine procedure used to improve appearance seems to be rapidly gaining ground. Obviously cosmetic surgery has an extremely important part to play in helping people who've suffered some kind of disfigurement. But people are now routinely subjecting themselves to surgical procedures in order to reduce the size of their tummy, increase the size of their breasts etc.. Inevitably some of those procedures will go wrong, there will be complications, and there may even be fatalities. So why do people do it? Why are they prepared to take the risk? I'm sure that a lot of the time people don't actually think very much about the risk as they have been lulled into a false sense of security. The 'it's amazing what they can do these days' and the almost everyday nature of surgery will no doubt have contributed to that. And then there's the pressure to be perfect. The media bombards us with images of perfect people and the perfect lifestyle. Maybe we are being pressured into expecting too much from life. Rather than being encouraged to be content with 'our lot' we are always being encouraged to make 'our lot' better. And we are constantly presented with ways in which we can improve our life: a better car, a more exotic holiday, cosmetic surgery, all will take us closer to the ideal, the dream. In doing so we forget that the key to our happiness lies within ourselves. Yes, if our car is old, noisy and unreliable then a new car will improve our quality of life, if we haven't had a holiday for awhile then time away will be beneficial, but how often are these things really needed?

Unfortunately, it's easier to think that the solution to our problems can be provided by external sources; that we can indeed buy into the dream. We need to stand back and take a good look at ourselves to see what the pressures are actually doing to us. By being constantly bombarded with images of the non existent perfect people and perfect lifestyles we are being made to feel dissatisfied with our life even when our life is good.

There have to be some bad times for everyone and we need to accept that. Bad things can happen to good people and however wrong it seems good things happen to bad people! When things are difficult the solution is not to buy something new. If we're not happy with our appearance the solution is not at the end of the surgeon's knife.

Chapter Six

Malignancy at 80mph?

When I relayed the news of my hospital visit to friends and family it was assumed by all that I would eventually have to have surgery. People had got used to the idea that for some strange reason I was going to delay treatment as long as possible, but they accepted the malignancy risk as both real and unacceptable and took it to mean I would have surgery. However I was not so sure as I had already searched once for evidence of the malignancy risk and failed to find any. It was obviously time to try again. I could not accept that if the risk was as great as implied by the Professor they would continue to use Gamma Knife so extensively in Sweden, but how could I find out?

For once luck was on my side. I'd joined the International Radiosurgery Support Association (then known as the International Gamma Knife Support Association) and in the next issue of the newsletter to drop through my letter box was an article by a physician who had trained at the Karolinska Institute in Stockholm. In the article he stated that he considered the risk of radiation causing malignancy to be 0.1%. The article also said which hospital in America he was now working in, so I faxed him to ask on what basis he had made that statement. He quickly replied stating that out of 3,000 patients he knew of 2 or perhaps 3 who developed malignant tumours. As Acoustic Neuromas are extremely rarely malignant anyway I considered that number to be inconclusive. But even if the risk was 0.1% that was still a lot better than the 1% risk of not surviving surgery.

When I next saw my GP he was completely bewildered. He read the letter from the Professor and commented that the Gamma Knife consultant had not mentioned any such risks. It seemed to me that it was the first time he had seen consultants disagree to such an extent and he was unsure what to make of it. He was certainly not alone in that!

I also joined a new newsgroup which was only for Acoustic Neuroma patients and from a member of the group heard of a new treatment called Fractionated Stereotactic Radiosurgery. In this treatment the radiation dose is delivered in 4 or 5 doses instead of one large one. My initial reaction was 'What a good idea! How sensible!' followed by another search of the medical research literature to see what I could find. Not a lot was the answer. My contact in America who was about to have the treatment at Staten Island University Hospital, New York sent me information, including some journal articles. The reported results looked very good; no facial nerve damage and almost 100% hearing preservation. It seemed such a logical treatment but I still couldn't believe what I was reading – if the reported results were accurate it seemed I may have finally found a 'treatment'! A procedure which could kill the tumour without risking devastating side effects! But of course being British my initial reaction was 'If something seems too good to be true then the chances are that it isn't'. So I faxed the American physician again to ask him what he thought of the treatment. He graciously replied that the results did indeed look very impressive and his only concern was whether or not the dose given was enough to kill the tumour. It is only now, many years later that I appreciate just how gracious and honest he was being. Medics tend to very much favour their own treatment and their own tradition and for him to express the opinion that an alternative treatment could be viable was rare indeed. I have never met him, but would like to.

The more I read my initial sceptical reaction was slowly replaced by a belief that this treatment might actually be the one for me, it might actually be what I had been searching for for so long.

Having found a possible treatment the big question was 'Is it available in the UK?' I'd discovered that the relocatable head frame was developed at a hospital in England so I emailed them to enquire about treatment there. Their response was 'Can't remember when we last treated an Acoustic Neuroma'. 'Oh dear' I thought 'the last thing I want is to go somewhere that doesn't normally treat the pesky things!'

Another holiday intervened, Easter, and we were to spend Easter weekend in Yorkshire. Little did I know as plans were made that the trip would be a turning point in the process. It seemed straightforward enough – someone we knew wanted to come to Wales for a few days so we were going to swop houses.

The journey there was mainly along motorways, which meant travelling at around 80 mph. OK I know that's over the official speed limit, but it does seem to be around the unofficial one! This journey was different though. After about 45 minutes my head began to feel weird, the pressure inside it was almost intolerable and just sitting in the car was a huge effort. The simple process of being a car passenger had suddenly become an enormous effort and it was an effort which my system couldn't cope with, so it simply switched off, I went to sleep. But it wasn't a pleasant sleep; even the sleep itself was tiring! By the time we arrived at our destination I felt as if I'd flown to Australia and had to go to bed to recover. That experience was a huge shock as previously long or short car journeys had not been a problem. They were in fact part of our lifestyle; camping holidays spent in the South of France involved very long journeys, much, much longer than across to Yorkshire. The only problems I'd been used to were how to keep babies and young children happy. Suddenly I had gone from being a good traveller to a person for whom just sitting in a car was an overwhelming effort! Why? Just what was that 'thing in my head' doing now?

As time went on the dull ache behind my ear spread and became an actual headache which on occasions became severe. The frequency of the severe headaches increased and the duration of them increased to. One day I woke and realised that I didn't have a headache, scarily the reason I noticed was because it was the first morning I'd woke without a headache for a week or more. When aches creep up like that it's amazing how they become part of life. The feeling of pressure had progressed so slowly to a headache that I hadn't noticed it doing so, and the frequency and intensity of the headaches had again increased so slowly that I hadn't noticed. But that morning I realised that I had to do something, my head was trying to tell me something, the headaches were bad. I was somehow accommodating them into my life but the quality of my life was diminishing rapidly.

I decided to contact Dr Lederman who carried out the treatment at Staten Island University Hospital and ask if he knew of anywhere in Britain which was doing the treatment. I sent him a fax and much to my amazement he phoned me within the hour! I was completely taken aback, so much so that I found it difficult to remember all of my questions. We discussed the treatment and he confirmed what I had read. He didn't know of anywhere in the UK, but then he said that his hospital had a special rate for people from overseas and the treatment might not be as expensive as I thought. Our perception is that medical treatment in America is prohibitively expensive and so I still assumed it would be far too much, but thought that I'd ask anyway. I was pleasantly surprised when he told me it would cost the equivalent of second hand car.

We'd actually been saving money for a new second hand car, so had that amount saved. A friend's sister worked for an airline so she could get very cheap standby tickets. For the cost of a 3 year old middle of the road car the treatment could be obtained. It was tempting.

I decided to give the hospital that had developed the headframe one last try and emailed them saying that Dr. Lederman had mentioned them. The reply this time was to emphasise the fact that they'd developed the head frame which he used, but as to Acoustic Neuroma their only comment was 'Microsurgery is the preferred treatment for Acoustic Neuroma in the UK'. 'Great' I thought 'guinea pig I am not!' and ruled out any possibility of treatment in the UK.

However, I still couldn't decide whether to go ahead with the treatment or not. I'd decided that the fractionated treatment offered at Staten Island was the best option available, but would it be better to carry on waiting? Maybe the tumour was not growing, maybe I could avoid treatment?

There seemed no answer to my question as I was not scheduled to have a scan for another few months and knew it would be very difficult to get it brought forward. But the symptoms were getting much worse. Even if the tumour was not growing it was doing something which was not good. My hearing was stable, and my facial nerve was still unaffected but the headaches were now a fact of life and were regularly bad, especially at night. Finding a comfortable pillow and working out the ideal number to use had become a major challenge. The wrong pillow and I woke up feeling as if my head was resting on a block of concrete. I also began to feel increasingly tired and it was an enormous effort to get through each day. Whether the tumour was growing or not had somehow become irrelevant. It was doing something which was not good – it would have to be treated.

Chapter Seven

Decision Time and The Pyrenees

Once I'd made the decision everything happened very quickly. I faxed Dr. Lederman who asked for my scans to be sent over. Copies of my hearing tests were also sent and within a month I had a phone call asking me when I would like to go over for the treatment. I was told that I could choose, as long as I didn't want treatment the following week!

By now it was late June and the school summer holidays were looming ahead. Some people thought I should go over straight away so that I could be back in time to enjoy the school holidays, but I wasn't so sure. I didn't know how I'd feel immediately after the treatment and I certainly didn't want to be away while the children were off school. So I decided to wait until the start of September. The appointment was duly made: Tuesday the 2nd of September, 10 am. I wrote the date in my diary and of course immediately worried that I hadn't done the right thing! The words looked so innocent on the page but I knew that they could change my life, perhaps for better, perhaps, ultimately, for the worse.

We'd planned an extensive camping holiday that year, crossing from Portsmouth to Bilbao in Northern Spain to spend a week in the Picos de Europa mountains, then a drive east for week in The Pyrenees, a slow drive up through France and finally a week in Brittany. By now I knew that motorway journeys were a problem and I was concerned about how I'd cope with the distances involved. My concern was justified, from the initial drive down to Portsmouth through to the final drive back up to North Wales they proved to be extremely difficult.

Somewhat inevitably I'd been having second thoughts about the treatment before the holiday but by the time we returned I had no doubt whatsoever that I was doing the right thing. Before going I wondered whether I wasn't exaggerating the symptoms, maybe it had stopped growing so I didn't need any treatment at all. That proved to be pure wishful thinking as there were many, many times when I felt so bad all I wanted to do was get on a plane and go back to wet and windy Wales. I love the sun and the Picos de Europa is one of the most beautiful and unspoilt regions of Europe I have ever visited but I felt too bad to appreciate it. And it wasn't just the long journeys. My head seemed to be permanently aching and bending down was agony. I discovered that one big problem of camping is the number of times it's necessary to bend down! But when I did it felt as if my brain was loose and it moved forward onto my forehead, causing severe pain as it did so. If I had to remain bent down for more than a few seconds I could hardly stand up again I felt so dizzy. Those effects surprised me, but the effects of the long motorway stretches did not. The only way to describe it is that my system shut down which then left me feeling exhausted and not just for the rest of the day, but the following day too.

Night times became worse as the holiday progressed. We'd bought a 'luxurious' folding camp bed for me but even so comfort for my head was difficult to find. By the final week I would wake every night feeling almost overwhelmed by a desire to get up and get out of the tent. The short ferry journey back added yet more weight to my decision. I was exhausted just sitting down. I looked for somewhere to lie down but even that was tiring, I was desperate to get off the boat, to simply stop moving.

So I returned from the holiday feeling totally exhausted but convinced that I had made the correct decision about having treatment. There were 2 weeks of the school holiday left and I spent them trying to rest as much as possible, and to take consolation from the fact that there was no motorway across the Atlantic! Flying could not be any worse than being on a motorway.

Eventually the departure day arrived and it felt very strange leaving the house at 5.30 in the morning to get to Heathrow for the plane. Part of me still did not want to go, but logic had prevailed. This was something which I didn't want to do but knew that I had to do. However much I hoped and wished otherwise the tumour had to be treated.

Some people were concerned because I was going over for treatment by myself, but I actually did not mind going alone. The search for treatment had been a lonely experience and I had grown accustomed to attending appointments by myself. It felt like a natural conclusion to finish by going for treatment by myself.

Chapter Eight

New York, New York

So 2 years 2 months after the first MRI I was on my way to New York. It had been an extremely difficult and frequently emotional journey, but I had made it. Strangely, I felt very little anxiety about having the treatment. After the holiday experiences I knew that I had to have treatment and I was confident that in the Fractionated Stereotactic Radiosurgery (FSR) offered by Gil Lederman I had found the most suitable treatment. The journey had been so difficult I was simply relieved that it was coming to an end. Looking back it is still the journey from initial MRI to treatment that I remember the most. My most vivid memories of New York and Staten Island are not the treatment memories, but memories of people and places. I'm sure the treatment is extremely difficult and complicated to plan and carry out, but as a patient I was blissfully unaware of that. Strange as it may seem, having the treatment proved to be the easy part, much, much easier than the 2 year journey that had taken me there.

I flew to New York at the end of August 1997, the day Diana, Princess of Wales was killed in the car crash. On the tube from Euston to Heathrow I caught a glimpse of a newspaper headline that read "Diana is Dead". For some reason that didn't actually register as I assumed it was not a literal statement, rather that she had behaved in an unacceptable way. Then before take off the pilot expressed his condolences to all British people on the plane and at that point I realised that she had indeed died.

The plane must have been very full on its return journey as it seemed that every American journalist had moved to London. I'd flown all the way across the Atlantic to see TV reporters standing in front of Buckingham Palace. The accent may have been different, but the location shots all looked very familiar. As you can imagine every time I spoke people wanted to know what my views on her death were and every taxi driver seemed to have an opinion on what had really happened in the tunnel. The only thing they had in common was that no-one seemed to think it was an accident.

The flight had been very comfortable, largely because of being able to fly 'connoisseur class', one of the perks of the buddy ticket. Having flown across the Atlantic in cattle class a few years previously I fully appreciated the difference. The extra space makes an enormous difference, and being in front of the engines means considerably less noise. Although I wasn't aware of it I understand that the air quality is better too. All of which meant that I arrived at Newark Airport feeling considerably better than if I had driven a couple of motorway hours into England.

Although New York is a popular tourist destination I doubt the same can be said for Staten Island. The hotel had at one time been a Holiday Inn and so looked the same as many other hotels. On one side ran an 8 lane highway and on the other was the fire station. Peace and quiet was not an option. But I wasn't there on holiday and the hotel was functional and clean. The situation may have been noisy but it was also convenient; the bus stopped right outside and there was a convenience store across the road. Coming from the UK, and especially coming from a rural area, so many things seemed strange. Every morning the news reported a shooting fatality yet when I asked for a bottle of wine in the convenience store the assistant looked surprised and told me I'd have to go to a liquor store for wine as they were only allowed to sell beer!

I'd allowed myself one day to recover from the journey and then it was time for my first appointment at the hospital. My first impression was how kind the staff were and how they seemed genuinely interested in people. Before the treatment could begin there were various tests to do and of course the fitting of the all important head frame. The first time I was asked 'And how are you paying for the treatment?' I thought it very bizarre as of course I'd never been asked before. I'd given a banker's draft to one of the finance people when I arrived so I simply had to state who I had given the draft to and they were happy. Some of my early experiences at the hospital were comical; their computer system was set up for American Zip Codes and so would not accept a UK postcode; in the word repetition section of my hearing test the greatest challenge was attempting to understand the tester's very heavy New York accent. The person operating the MRI scanner was interested to know what kind of machines we had in the UK, big, cold and noisy didn't seem to be enough detail for her.

Other experiences were very moving. I remember being in the waiting room and a man sat down next to me while the patient he was with was taken to a different room. I commented that his friend looked very ill and he must be very concerned about him. The reply shocked me as although both men looked to be in their early fifties they were actually father and son; the son had a malignant brain tumour. I don't know but I can't imagine that the son survived, I suspect the treatment was palliative.

In a direct contrast to my consultations with the professor in the UK Gil Lederman was very easy to talk to and discuss things with. He asked if I wanted to speak to any previous patients, we discussed how far apart to space the treatments and he explained how they ensured that the head frame was located in the precise place for each treatment. He knew that I'd travelled by myself and to my surprise he gave me his out of hours contact number, with the instruction to not hesitate to phone if I was concerned about anything. I never needed to use it, but just knowing I had a contact number was very re-assuring.

We discussed at length how far apart to space the treatments and decided to have 5 treatment sessions mostly on alternate days, but to have two on consecutive days to avoid having to spend another weekend on Staten Island. During the discussion I was struck again by how logical the treatment was, and I wondered again just why it had been so difficult for me to find it.

On a couple of my 'days off' I caught the famous Staten Island ferry and sailed by the Statue of Liberty to Manhattan. I'd heard people comment before that visiting Manhattan is very strange because even if you've never been before it's so familiar from films that you feel like you've already seen it. I found that to be so true. I went into a diner for lunch and was amazed to see a couple of policeman sitting at the bar drinking their coffee, just like they do in the films! They really do sit with their guns and coffee apparently doing nothing more than passing the time of day. And steam from the subway really does come through gratings in the pavement! After being used to the underground in London which descends way way below the surface I was taken aback by how close to the surface the New York subway was.

On treatment days my routine was different. To the horror of one of the female physicists I'd catch the bus to the hospital. She was concerned because the bus went through less desirable parts of Staten Island and I had to change busses at one point, but it was mid morning and it seemed fine. The change of bus corner would probably have been rather scary later in the day though. I quite enjoyed the journeys as I saw a side of Staten Island that I would never have seen from a taxi. A couple of mornings the same teenager caught the bus, presumably late for school, and promptly fell asleep again. Somehow he managed to wake up in time for his stop. Another day an evangelical lady sat next to me and gave me her personal views on the bible for a good half hour.

After treatment I would take a taxi back to the hotel. The bus route and taxi route couldn't have been more different though. The taxi took the direct route and went through leafy suburbs of large detached houses with extensive manicured lawns and, of course, no pavement. Again, it was very reminiscent of countless movies and I couldn't help but observe that the taxi route was the image most frequently portrayed in films. The bus route was severely neglected by the media; small terraced houses with tiny front gardens and small run down shops.

The treatment itself was well planned and painless. The headframe was located by means of a dental mould and various straps. It had taken an entire afternoon to set up. For each treatment session depth readings were taken when it was put in place and a second person came in specifically to check the readings were accurate. The back of the frame was attached to the couch for treatment and although the rest of me could move my head was very much in one place, and reassuringly so. Before delivering the radiation the staff obviously left the room and I was left alone while the machine moved above my head. I knew that the radiation was potentially very dangerous but I felt absolutely nothing; I couldn't see it, hear it, touch it or smell it.

I flew home the day after the final treatment session, feeling rather nauseous but otherwise OK. Compared to the difficulties of obtaining information and deciding on which treatment to have actually having the treatment was so very simple. People have frequently asked if I wasn't scared being by myself so far away from home - I wasn't, not in the slightest.

The following weeks I was incredibly tired but then after about 3 months I noticed that my headaches had faded considerably and things just steadily improved after that. Slowly but surely I could feel that my health was improving, and reassuringly I noticed no sign of any facial nerve problems and my hearing remained the same.

Even so I was very concerned when it was time to have the first scan twelve months later. What if the tumour had continued to grow? Although I was concerned I also knew that the symptoms were considerably less and continuing to diminish, which I hoped meant that the scan would reveal nothing untoward, and it didn't. Whilst waiting for it I had a few interesting conversations with myself. A few people asked if I would have surgery if the scan revealed that the tumour had grown. I never answered their question with anything other than a 'cross that bridge if I come to it' kind of answer.

In conversation with myself I tried to honestly answer the 'what if it's grown' question. I never did manage to decide what I would do if it had, because, thankfully, the question has never needed answering. But I did answer the 'would you ever regret having FSR' question. And the answer was 'no I would not'. It's something of a cliché to say 'all we can ever do is make the best decision that we can at the time', but like a lot of clichés it's also true. And I had actually **made** a decision; I hadn't just taken the easy way out. Unfortunately I can think of many other occasions when taking the easy way out was all I had done. So I think the cliché really needs to be elaborated: all we can do is make the best decision we can with the evidence available at the time. But we must actually make our own decision, after all it's our life so we should take responsibility for it.

It's now 10 years since the treatment and things have continued to go well. I have no damage to the facial nerve; have hearing in two ears and can conduct a phone conversation with the affected ear if I have to.

And I still can't sing in tune.

Fractionated Stereotactic Radiosurgery

I realise that some people may be disappointed that I didn't include more details about the treatment. Although it may seem strange actually having the treatment was the easiest part of the whole process, so rather than me trying to explain what is a complicated procedure I think it's best if people look at Gil Lederman's website (www.rsny.org).

On the website the treatment is described in varying detail, for the most detail I suggest following the 'Questions asked by European patients' link.

The rapid growth of the internet and the world wide web means that anyone with access to it is unlikely to have the same protracted search for information that I experienced. However, although information can now be readily found the problem of interpreting the information, dealing with friends and family, and making decisions remains.

Good Luck.

www.ingramcontent.com/pod-product-compliance
Lightning Source LLC
Chambersburg PA
CBHW050556280326
41933CB00011B/1861